CLEFT PALATE AND SPEECH